Essential Oils Reference Guide for Healthy Skin

How to Use Essential Oils to Cure Acne, Remove Scars, Achieve Smooth Skin

By

Erika Robinson

Essential Oils Reference Guide for Healthy Skin

First edition. May, 2018.

Copyright © 2018 Erika Robinson

Written by Erika Robinson

Table of Contents

Introduction

The skin, the biggest and largest organ, and one of the most important organs in the body, is the first immune system of man; it interconnects with the environment and protects the internal organs and tissues of the body from germs and excessive loss of water.

It has important roles and functions which it carries out. It even helps in the elimination of waste products and toxins; that is why it is sometimes called the "third kidney".

This organ is used in the diagnosis of diseases; it regulates body temperature, and supports the sensation of cold, touch, pain and heat. The skin is the seat for the sixth and most delicate sense, touch.

It helps in the circulation of blood and regulation of blood pressure; it can repair itself, it cleanses itself, it is a respiratory organ, and it is an acidic barrier that stops the invasion of germs and parasites.

It is a known and ignored fact that we need to take care of our skin to keep it healthy. When the skin is neglected, it can result to skin problems like rashes, eczema, dermatitis, acne, dandruff, psoriasis, rosacea, cellulite, skin abscess, skin cancer, melanoma, warts, hives, seborrheic keratosis, scabies, shingles, ringworm, etc.

Causes of skin problems and infections are bad diet, unhealthy lifestyle, malnutrition, dehydration, smoking, stress, excessive drinking, exposure to germs, toxins and harmful rays, untreated skin infections and wounds etc.

Essential oils?

There are numerous ways to take care of the skin; hydration is the most important, intake of healthy foods, exercise, relaxation and treatment with essential oils.

Essential oils are concentrated oils gotten from parts of medicinal plants and herbs; they are usually hydrophobic and volatile and are mostly used for therapeutic purposes.

Essential oils are also used on the skin for many purposes; some of them are to protect the skin from harmful rays and sunburn, to keep the skin healthy, to treat skin problems and infections, to brighten the skin and make it glow, they inhibit prevent pre-mature aging, clear the signs of aging and prevent skin cancer.

Essential Oils Good for The Skin

Carrot seed essential oil: It rejuvenates the skin; it fights premature aging and clears signs of aging like wrinkles and fine lines, it makes the skin smooth and enhances the process of cell regeneration.

It has a rich amount of antioxidants; it fights inflammation, it fades scars and prevents the formation and activities of free radicals.

Basil essential oil: This oil is best for people with sensitive skin; it hastens wounds healing and prevents infection and skin problems. It is even used in the treatment of insect bites and treats other skin issues.

Rosehip seed oil: Extracted from the seeds of rose bushes; this is one of the strongest fighter of aging; it is rich in antioxidants that protects the skin from damage.

It clears spots, brighten complexion, smoothen skin and clears aging signs.

Neroli essential oil: This oil is best for oily skin, sensitive and mature skin; it clears fine lines and wrinkles, it restores sagging skin and prevents rapid aging.

It can regenerate the skin due to its rich content of Citral; it can effectively remove stretch marks, red marks and prevents them from forming in the first place.

It also has antiseptic properties which prevent skin infections caused by germs and it regulates the production of oil thereby preventing acne breakout.

It unblocks pores and does not cause skin wilting.

Marula essential oil: This oil is effective in preventing acne breakout and it fades the scars; it is derived from the nuts of Africa marula tree, it is loaded with antibacterial properties, it normalizes the levels of hormones and do not block the pores.

Lemongrass essential oil: This oil can effectively treat stubborn acne and large skin pores; it is an effective skin toner, it enhances the look of the skin and gives it a natural glow.

It is packed full with astringent properties. It repels bugs and protects the skin.

Sesame seed essential oil: It is rich in essential fatty acids like palmitic acid, oleic acid, stearic acid and linoleic acid. This helps to keep the skin hydrated, supple and it also increases blood flow and circulation.

It reverses cellulite, stretch marks and other scars on the skin.

Frankincense essential oil: This oil effectively treats dry skin, skin problems and it can be used by any skin type. It clears acne and skin blemishes; it stops pre-mature aging, it reduces scarring and treats dry skin.

It is good for acne-prone skin and oily skin; it has antimicrobial and anti-inflammatory properties; it tones the skin, decrease pore size and gives the skin an even complexion.

It boosts the production of new skin cells; enhances the growth of new cells, it tightens the skin, clears wrinkles and scars and soothes a dry and chapped skin.

Camellia seeds essential oil: This oil is rich in Omega-6 and omega-9; this makes the skin soft and moisturized, it does not leave a greasy residue when applied on the skin, it is good in controlling dry skin.

Cypress essential oil: This oil is good at repairing damaged skin; it also repairs damaged capillaries and veins around the nose, it shrinks swollen blood vessels and closes the pores of the skin.

Lemon balm essential oil: This minty oil is rich in antioxidants like ferulic acid and caffeine; these expel toxins, protect the skin against harmful rays and toxins. It boosts hydration and prevents reduction of moisture.

Patchouli essential oil: This is one of the best remedies for aging; it boots growth of new skin cells, it clears wrinkles and fine lines and makes the appearance of the skin smooth.

It has antimicrobial and antiseptic properties; it protects the skin from infections and problems like dermatitis, acne, eczema and psoriasis.

Bergamot essential oil: This oil is rich in natural antiseptic properties; it kills microbes that can cause skin problems, it hastens wound healing and repairs damaged skin.

It can be applied directly to eczema, acne scars and psoriasis for quick healing and to fade the scars.

Juniper essential oil: This is a powerful cleansing oil; it eliminates dirt, germs and dead skin cells from the surface of the skin and gives it a natural glow.

It hastens the healing of wounds and it can effectively treat wound infections due to its antimicrobial and antiseptic properties.

Moringa essential oil: This oil is gotten from Moringa seeds and it helps to fight dull appearance and it improves the appearance and glow of the skin.

It gives the skin a gorgeous look and a rosy glow; it fights rapid aging and skin fatigue, it refreshes the skin and gives one a radiant complexion.

Geranium essential oil: This oil is good for skin prone to acne; it controls the production of oil and thereby prevent acne breakout. It treats acne and other skin blemishes like dermatitis and eczema; it prevents rapid aging; it is good for dry skin.

It increases the elasticity of the skin; it closes the pores of the skin and tightens it, it reduces wrinkles on the skin and improves the flow of blood to areas it is applied on.

It is used in the treatment of wounds and bruises; it heals damaged capillaries, it heals burns, cuts, ringworm, eczema, and other skin problems.

Sunflower seed oil: Vey rich in vitamin E, this oil is a heavy-duty body hydrator; it nourishes the body and keeps it hydrated. It treats dry skin.

Chamomile essential oil: This oil is used widely to treat lots of skin problems and conditions; it is effective against cracked feet, rosacea, chapped skin, acne, sensitive skin, inflammation and eczema.

Rosemary essential oil: This oil clears the surface of the skin of dead cells; it stimulates regeneration and fights dull appearance. It removes dead skin cells and reveals fresh ones underneath.

It is even applied on the scalp to treat scalp problems like dandruff and itchy scalp.

Rose essential oil: This is great natural remedy for dry and aging skin; it is rich in therapeutic compounds that heal wounds, infections and skin diseases.

It also has antimicrobial and anti-inflammatory properties which keeps skin infections and problems at bay; it enhance skin texture and skin tone, and it even prevents dehydration.

Clary essential oil: This oil is best at improving the genera; appearance of the skin; it fights aging and clears the signs of aging; it reduces puffiness and regulates oil production thereby preventing acne.

Eucalyptus oil: This oil is good for skin irritation and inflammation; it treats acne, treats wounds, cuts and bruises. It prevents scalp problems and increases blood flow to the hair; thereby improving its appearance and growth.

Lavender essential oil: Every lady shouldn't be without this; it even has a sweet sent and can be used as a natural perfume. It is good for oily skin and dry skin; it fights aging and reduce scarring.

It relieves stress and helps the body to relax; it helps the skin cells to regenerate, and it is effective against sunburn and sun spots. Lavender essential oil is recommended for the treatment of skin ailments and to provide the natural smoothness, which is very important even as it gives the sweet aroma.

Blue tansy oil: Rich in anti-inflammatory properties; this oil helps in preventing skin problems; it hydrates the skin, improve the complexion and makes it even.

Helichrysum essential oil: Also called "immortelle" because of effective way it combats aging and even reverses it; it is used in making natural anti-aging products.

It functions at the cellular level; it restores the structures of the cells and this fights cell aging. Though it is expensive; this is one of the best choices in fight aging.

Tea tree essential oil: This is the best oil for acne-prone skin; its powerful antibacterial properties keeps acne at bay and it hasten the healing of wound and prevents wound infections.

It regulates the production of oil and this helps in preventing acne breakout.

Myrrh essential oil: Is potent against blemish and oily skin; it is good for dry skin and it reduces the signs of aging, it erases scars and fight inflammation.

It improves skin firmness; skin tone, it improves the elasticity of the skin, reduces fine lines and wrinkles; it heals sunburns, rashes, eczema and chapped skin.

Pomegranate seed oil: This oil is used by naturopaths to treat skin cancer; it can be used as a natural skin serum and it has been used to treat skin problems since historic times.

It is a powerful fighter of rapid or premature aging; it has bioflavonoids that protect the skin from sun damage. Recently, pomegranate seed oil has been used rampantly as a natural sunscreen and also sunburn treatment ointment.

Ylang-ylang essential oil: This oil has a rich fragrance; it prevents the breakout of acne by controlling the production of oil, it helps to regenerate skin cells.

It prevents rapid aging and clears signs of aging like fine lines, age spots and wrinkles; it also boosts the elasticity of the skin and it can be used on the three skin types.

Argan oil: Made from the kernels of argan trees, this oil is rich in vitamin E and essential fatty acids and proteins which help in improving the health and appearance of the skin.

It hydrates the skin and strengthens it; it even helps brittle or weak nails and improves complexion and general

appearance.

Carrier Oils

Carrier Oils to Mix with Essential Oils:

Jojoba oil: This is one of best oils for hydrating the skin; it moisturizes the skin without leaving an oily appearance.

"Jojoba oil has been used widely around the world as a skin moisturizer because of its properties of attracting moisture. Most importantly, it traps moisture and keeps the skin moisturized for a significantly long period of time."

Additionally, jojoba oil is rich in vitamins, which are vital for healthy and nourished skin.

Natural moisturizing is one of jojoba oil's known qualities. This does not mean that the oil keeps the skin oily, but it gets rid of excess oil and therefore keeps the skin soft and shiny. On the other hand, keeping the skin texture at a natural level helps in the prevention of acne. People have used jojoba oil to remove acne scars, skin roughness and to stop skin irritation.

Apricot oil:

Very rich in vitamin A and E; this oil is very gentle on skin. It has the property of nourishing the skin effectively. Modern mothers have discovered the magic of apricot oil recently and have been using the essential oil on kids' skin. It provides just the mild action and health benefits at the same time. people with sensitive skin can also use apricot oil to provide the needed soothing feeling.

Grapeseed oil: This is a common ingredient in many anti-aging serums and body creams because of its ability to restore the elasticity of the skin.

It makes the skin firm; erases fine lines and restores collagen. It is rich in polyphenols which fight inflammation.

Almond oil: This oil is rich in omega-3 fatty acids; it keeps the skin soft, hydrated and gives it a natural glow. It is hypoallergenic and can be used on irritated and sensitive skin; it treats skin problems like psoriasis and eczema.

Avocado oil: This oil is rich in healthy fats which make the skin glow; it hydrates the skin and stimulates the production of collagen. It is a better alternative for skin serum that is loaded with chemicals.

Coconut oil: This oil improves the health of the skin and it is great for dry skin; it keeps the skin moist, hydrated and prevents loss of moisture, it is a gentle makeup remover and it prevents bacterial infections.

Olive oil: This oil is good in treating skin problems; it is even effective against itchy scalp, and dandruff. It is rich in

antibacterial and antifungal compounds;
it treats sunburns and protects the skin
from damages.

How to Use Essential Oils

Essential oils have been used since pre-historic times for skin care and other health benefits; please ensure you go for high quality essential oils, make sure they are pure and free from contamination.

Dilute essential oils; it is critical.

When you want to apply essential oil directly on the skin; it is advisable to mix them with carrier oil. This is because these oils have very high concentrations of the healing phytochemicals of the plant they were extracted from. This can be poisonous; excessive dose of good things is also bad.

It can even cause reaction for sensitive skin; when applied directly it can cause skin irritations and burns. They can even cause skin sensitization; this can lead to a permanent allergic response and can make it impossible for you to ever use that oil again. So to avoid all these; it is advisable you mix any essential oil you want to use with a cold pressed carrier oil.

Carrier oils are mentioned above; choose one that you like most and use it to dilute an essential oil you choose to use. When using it on your whole body; it is best to mix one part of essential oil with 2 parts of carrier oil.

If you want to apply it on a specific skin part; then you will need a little quantity of the essential oil; in this case you can dilute two drops of the essential oil with one teaspoon of carrier oil, this mixture can be applied directly on an affected skin part.

Mixing equal parts of essential oil and carrier oil is not advisable unless it is done under the supervision of a trained health professional.

Carrier oils are also beneficial and have their own therapeutic effects; they make the essential oil more effective and powerful. Another reason why you need to dilute your essential oil with carrier oils is that carrier oils prevent them from evaporating.

Essential oils are volatile; when applied on the skin without mixing, they will evaporate and this will affect its potency and effectiveness. Carrier oils are complemented with essential oil by means of mixing, in order to help the essential oil to penetrate deep into your skin.

It is not advisable to ingest essential oil except stated otherwise by herbalist or a doctor; and it must be mixed with a carrier oil before taking it orally so that it will not irritate the mouth and esophagus.

Note that it is possible to mix more than two essential oils together; it is called oil blending and it is great way to maximize the health benefits of these oils. You can even mix the best oils for your skin types or when you are having more than one skin condition, like fighting aging and sensitive skin at the same time.

You must mix this oil blend with carrier oil too. Put your oil blend in amber colored bottles; this will protect the oils from direct rays of light. Pregnant women and infants are to avoid some essential oils; so do your research before

using any.

Application of Essential Oils

You can directly apply them on the skin

When you've created your oil blend and properly mixed it with a carrier oil; you can apply this mixture on your whole body or to a specific skin part depending on what you want.

You can also use it to massage your body. This increases the flow of blood to the skin; boosts appearance and relieve stress.

Soaking

Another way to benefit from essential oils is by adding them to your bath water and soak in it for at most 20 minutes; add at least 10 drops of an essential oil to your regular bath water, when blending two oils, add five drops each. The number of drops should reduce as the number of oils increase.

This gives the skin a unique glow, relieve stress, and shield the skin from bacterial infections and fades scars.

Face cleanse

A face cleanse also known as oil cleanse is an effective way to moisturize your skin and keep the signs of aging at bay. It reverses dull skin, saggy skin, and keeps the face youthful.

You can do a face cleanse twice daily, once daily, many times weekly or once a week; this depends on what you are trying to achieve. A face cleanse is easy to do.

•	Get warm water and use it to wash your face; this will unclog and free the pores.

•	Take your mixture (your essential oil diluted with carrier oil) and massage your face with it for at most two minutes. Make sure you touch every part of your face and it should be done in an upward rotation way.

•	Let the mixture sit on the face for at least 1 minute.

- Dip a clean cloth or soft water in warm water and squeeze lightly.

- Place the towel on your face for 30 seconds.

- Then you use it to wipe your face; do this slowly and gently.

- Dip the towel in warm water again and repeat the cleaning process till you feel your face is clean enough.

- Then you splash cold water on your face to close the pores and send blood rushing to the face; it will also give

your face a natural glow.

Skin Types and Essential Oils

Skin types and the essential oils best for them

Those with oily skin who want to reduce the production of oil can use the following essential oils.

They are Cypress, orange, geranium, lemon, bergamot, and lime essential oils.

Those with dry and chapped skin can use German or Roman chamomile, cedarwood, palmarosa, geranium, sandalwood, and myrrh essential oils.

People with combination skin types can use orange, patchouli, bergamot and lavender essential oils.

Essential Oils and Skin Conditions

Essential oils for specific skin conditions:

For skin breakouts and blemishes; you can use tea tree, patchouli, geranium, lavender, and vetiver essential oils. To clear stubborn spots; you can apply them undiluted on the spot.

To reverse aging and put a stop to rapid or premature aging; you can make use of these oils:

Elemi,

Tangerine,

Sandalwood,

Palmarosa,

Ylang-ylang,

Rose,

Patchouli,

Frankincense

Lavender

Cypress essential oils.

In order to get rid of red marks, scars or spots, use the following essential oils:

*   Lemon essential oils.

*   Lavender

*   Frankincense

The effectiveness of these oils on the skin is highly significant.

To avoid photosensitivity: Note that some essential oils can lead to photosensitivity; examples are citrus essential oils and some other types, they lead to photosensitivity when used on the skin and you expose that part to sunlight.

It makes the individual susceptible to irritation, redness and burning; dilute the oils properly and it will be advisable to use them at night.

Essential oils that can cause photosensitivity are bergamot, German chamomile, grapefruit, cinnamon, lime, rue, lemon, angelica, orange and ginger essential oils.

www.ingramcontent.com/pod-product-compliance
Lightning Source LLC
Chambersburg PA
CBHW070049260726
48658CB00002B/814